ME, MYSELF AND OCD

AN EXPERIENCE THROUGH MENTAL HEALTH

By: Sean Bell

DISCLAIMER

TRIGGER WARNING.

TABLE OF CONTENTS

INTRODUCTION

This book is about my journey through mental health and how I have coped with it over several years. You will be able to have an insight into my journey and some of the hurdles that I have overcome, to be able to give you this book to read today. The main goal of writing this book is to raise awareness and show that you are not alone in these trying times.

Throughout my life, I set out to find personal experiences like mine, but with difficulty, as there aren't many, and all I did find was that I had to read a lot of different books and articles to begin to accumulate some ideas for what it was I was experiencing. As you might imagine, doing so while feeling smothered and overwhelmed by my thinking was difficult. By writing this, I hope to ease that pain and make your recovery easier. What you are going to read is a mixture of insights into feelings and symptoms around specific mental health experiences but also tied with my opinion as my journey has often been frustrating and scary.

I feel that my suffering over a decade of numerous mental health symptoms and my experience through innumerable therapies and research is enough to give helpful information to others that may be experiencing similar. The context in this book will help you understand what you may be feeling and provide you with methods that I used to deal with specific situations. I aim to help you understand and build awareness.

CHAPTER ONE: WHERE IT ALL STARTED

Before we dive into my mental health journey, I would like to give you a little insight into my younger years, which seems a lifetime ago, even at 30 years of age.

Like many other young kids, my upbringing was unsettled as my parents got divorced. Unbeknown to a younger me, this created a lot of uncertainty in my life at a young age. I was a young boy crying for a father who had left much to his choosing. At this age, I was very unaware of my mentality and how this affected me, and along with my lack of experience and knowledge, this seemed 'normal'.

However, I had a loving and caring mother and a sister who used to like dressing me up and calling me 'Rosie'. My grandad was a 'tough man that I looked up to, partly because I feared him and the majority as a role model. To think in this generation that anybody mentioned mental health to my Grandad, I am certain I know what his response would be. Maybe something along the lines of 'Get a grip' or pull yourself together or maybe even 'shut up talking daft', which is almost what I still see in the world today.

As a youngster, I was very sensitive, and I was a mummy's boy,' which is why I was tormented so early in school. This changed me as a person, and I wouldn't even say I switched my personality and morals. It overtook them.

Many teenagers go through the same, as school life for numerous kids isn't the easiest. Like others, I changed and became one of the 'cool kids. I never really bullied anyone, but at the same time, I never stepped in to stop the bullies because I was trying to fit in, so I didn't become the next target. I did things as a teenager that I am ashamed of when I look back due to changing myself to feel like I fit into society. This became a problem during recovery, and as we go through this book, you will see how apparent that becomes.

My early childhood isn't that important, but I feel a sharp insight into the sort of upbringing I had as a boy and the environment which surrounded me will help you understand the extra hurdle and difficulty that comes when dealing with mental health when you didn't really 'know yourself because you changed to fit in with society.

CHAPTER TWO: THE TRAUMA

There are wounds on the body that never show up on the surface that are deeper and more painful than anything that bleeds."

My story begins with my first baby, Blake. Blake was born on the 26th of April 2012 and was overdue by two weeks, and the pregnancy was smooth sailing, although I am pretty sure my wife would disagree. What I mean by smooth sailing is that there were no complications, issues, or abnormalities, and as far as everyone knew, Blake would be excellent when he arrived with us. However, an immature mind with minimal life experience wouldn't be aware of any dangers or life-changing events that we were about to go through.

Blake was born in our local hospital with no issues through birth. As a very first-time Dad, I was petrified. Even just trying to cut the umbilical cord seemed overwhelming to me. Nothing seemed real.

As time went on in the early morning after the birth, I was advised that I had to leave because my wife and Blake had to go up to the maternity ward, and it wasn't within the visiting hours, so I left. Around three hours later, my wife phoned me, and it became pretty apparent that something wasn't right. She told me in tears that our newborn son had been rushed up to the Neonatal ward as he had a seizure when the doctors did the walk-around checks. I ran to the hospital to find tubes and wires attached to my newborn son, which was very alarming.

As you can imagine, we were scared and frustrated to not have any answers to why and what had happened because we just wanted him to be okay, to take him home so that we could go and live the life that we had planned within the nine months of my wife carrying him.

Over the next 10 days, Blake didn't improve, and we soon found the news that we never expected to hear... "there is nothing we can do for him". This still hurts and sticks even 10 years later, and we were distraught. Blake was diagnosed with NKH (Non-Ketotic Hyperglycinemia), a genetic disorder, which meant that he didn't have the metabolic to break down protein in his body. A buildup of protein becomes toxic and soon impacts the brain, effectively damaging the brain to the point of no recovery. We had no option but to turn off the life support machine and watch our beautiful ten-day-old son leave us, this was absolutely devastating, and no words can describe the feeling of a loss like this. Blake was buried on the 21st of May 2012.

After the death of our son, we were offered bereavement, but we were young and naïve. We weren't aware of mental health back then. What even was it? We were never told how it might impact any of us, and we turned it down, not knowing what was happening or what had just happened. I point this out because when I think back, I think, should I have tried it?

Later in the year 2012, I was diagnosed with depression as all I wanted to do was die. My life was empty, and I felt I had nothing to live for, and all I wanted to do was withdraw from society and sleep my life away. I hid for three months in a bedroom;

I withdrew from people around me and just threw myself into video games to pass the time. I lost all my motivation, ambition, and sense of belonging. The trauma I was suffering or suffered from absolutely destroyed me!

The In between

After my three months of hibernation in 2012, I sought some motivation from deep in and had some fire in my belly, and I stood up in the hole I allowed myself to creep into. I thought this wasn't a life I wanted, so I chose to stand up to what seemed to be a 'silent killer. I switched all my focus onto a career as I knew there would be some advantages to the new journey I was about to lead. I went back to college and finished my qualification to get more money. I was young and had a lot of hunger back to fight for a better life. However, the mental habits I got through this time would be a life changer as we go through the rest of this journey.

In 2013, the year after Blake's death, my now-wife fell pregnant with my eldest daughter. It was a very challenging time given what we had just been through, but at the same time to other people, it felt like a blessing in disguise. I was very scared when I found out; my initial response wasn't one I like to look back on. When she was born, I found it very challenging to grow a bond with her. You would imagine I would have embraced this, but it turned out quite the opposite, and I struggled. It's like I had a barrier up, and mentally I wouldn't allow myself to care for other people or even show any signs of love as if it would resemble weakness. This was me now.

I was very selfish through these years, and my family always stood by me. I didn't show my wife that I cared for her. Well, I didn't show anyone I cared for them. We lived like this for years. I concentrated on work and progressing career-wise while leaving my wife to do the family part. In 2017, my youngest daughter was born. Again, I didn't really allow myself to bond with her, and I say really because I bonded with her a little bit more than what I did with my eldest daughter, but that affected relationships. It killed me inside.

Still, I could see that my eldest was noticing this bond between me and my youngest and maybe questioning why I wasn't like that with her.

After years of battling through jobs and different roles to become as good as I could be as an engineer, I felt that I was becoming emptier, like I was running out of things to achieve career-wise. I started as an apprentice, became independent as an engineer, and went into supervisory roles managing other people. The age I was at and the experience I had gained had put me in a position where I was competent at my job. I chucked myself into anything and everything. The problem is, the further I got, the less I felt I had to focus on. It became very apparent that I abandoned my personal life after Blake's death.

I have a best friend that would always question me on what he could see over the years, and he would say things like "when are you going to settle down?" or "another hobby again?". He could see I was bouncing in and out of things over the years, and he could see that I wasn't settled. I was always looking for the next thing to focus on or the next target and goal to hit. If I carried on and the opportunities came along, I would be the CEO of a global company by the time I was 35, but realistically, in life, that doesn't happen. It was easy for me to talk to him about this because he knew a lot about me.

Everything up to now should give you an excellent idea of what sort of person I was growing up, how I changed at school, the early part of becoming an adult, and the effect it had on myself and my relationships with others around me.

CHAPTER THREE: THE LIFE CHANGER

One night in December 2019, my wife and I were watching TV in bed, and it was no different from any other night over the years. We were watching a police documentary on our local TV station. It was no different to the types of programs we would watch any other time, we weren't into one category or niche, but we would give anything a watch, so this wasn't out of the ordinary, but it was this moment when everything changed for me.

This documentary covered a criminal case involving a murder which was caused by a stabbing. As the program went on, I could feel myself becoming more anxious/scared. Still, I didn't read too much into it as I had this sometimes when I watched something that involved something uncomfortable and immorally wrong. My wife and I both smoke, so as we would have a cigarette before bed, we went downstairs, my wife was already in the kitchen as I walked down, and as soon as I turned and glanced into the kitchen from the bottom of the stairs, I had a flashing image or a flashing thought that appeared as a movie scene in my mind about my wife being stabbed. This scared me so much that I tried to forget about it, but because I was trying to forget about it, my anxiety was increasing.

Further, every second felt like a minute, like an hour, and when I stood at the front door, my body went into full panic mode. The thought suppression I was trying to do was like trying to push a big inflatable beach ball underwater, and it just kept popping back up and hitting me in the face. All my body was shaking. It felt like everything in my body was just going to hit the floor, and all this was whilst my wife was standing at the side of me, not knowing that anything was wrong and, of course, 'IM NOT GOING TO TELL HER!

Why would I?

She might think I want to do it, or I'm going crazy for thinking such things like this. We went back upstairs after I had tried calming myself down, and I put something funny on the TV to go to sleep and distract myself from what had just happened to me.

The problem became bigger the next day. I got up around 6 am, got ready for work as normal, got in my van and headed up the motorway to my first job, which was around one and a half hours drive away. Within half an hour of driving, things started returning to me from last night, making me instantly anxious. Again, the more I tried not to think, the more they came, the bigger they became, the more powerful they became, and I couldn't get rid of them. All that was going around in my head was, 'why did you think that?' What does this mean to you? Does this mean you want to do it? Does this mean you're a killer? What if you do it? 'You're going to go to prison!' 'You don't deserve her' Why would you want to kill her?

I had these thoughts flying around my head along with images of every thought I was having, and as you can imagine, my anxiety skyrocketed, and when I got to my job, I couldn't even get out of my van because I was that scared and anxious! I was scared someone would hurt me or take me away for these thoughts, and I was scared that I might do something I didn't want to do! I didn't know what was happening to me.

Whilst at work, I messaged my wife and told her everything, and I told her I was very scared. Even though I didn't react, I just had to tell someone. Otherwise, I was going to end it all. When I got home and told my wife, I felt relief that she knew, but it didn't end the guilt, the shame, the severely high anxiety state, the loneliness. I needed answers for this!

I first found myself seeking reassurance from people, for them to say, 'you wouldn't do anything like that or 'I've had the same thoughts. It was like people were scared to admit anything, or maybe they didn't have them like me. But, at the same time, as much as I wanted someone to say I couldn't or wouldn't do anything like that for reassurance, I knew that wasn't reality deep down, which made it worse for me. Anyone can do anything in any given situation, which was a truth that made it worse! The unknown scared me even more!

Over the next few days, I got worse, and my anxiety level went up and up. I was restless, I was banging my head against the wall, and I was crying. I was distraught that this had happened to me, and I needed answers for what it was. What has happened to me? Why has it happened to me? Nobody had answers for me!

Every day just became a world of spinning thoughts that I would seem to be in rumination to, digging deep into the thought to find out what it meant or trying to find some relief in them. The problem is, is that this is the problem. Rumination is what keeps these thoughts powerful. It's what keeps them coming, making them bigger. But this seems real to me?!

I spoke to my best friend, and although he didn't have answers for me, he listened, he understood me, but again, the reassurance only lasted for a short while before it all started again!

I knew this was becoming out of control, and I sought out some sort of help from the NHS in the UK. It wasn't the easiest. I contacted the crisis team for mental health because all my doctor wanted to throw me some tablets, which I knew wouldn't help me in this situation. When I spoke to the crisis team, the person didn't catch on and understand what I was saying. I didn't feel any way; this triggered my anxiety and scared me even more.

I felt I was very vulnerable and sensitive to anything at that point. With anything said, my anxiety level was as high as it could be, and I would avoid everything that may make me worse. They made me an appointment at the hospital for an assessment.

I explained everything when I arrived and went into a room with my wife and the mental health nurse! She looked at me in a way where I didn't feel like she understood me, what I was going through, or what had happened to me! My confidence was shot. I didn't know what was going to happen next! I was scared I would get sectioned and lose everything I had worked for.

Of course, when you speak to any mental health professional, they always start with a statement that says, ' if we think you're a risk to yourself or anyone else, then we can break confidentiality'. If you're not anxious or scared about these thoughts alone, having someone say something like that will get you up there.

I came away from here with them telling me they would refer me to the mental health service for therapy, but this wasn't enough for me! I needed help there and then! Over the next few days, I went off sick from work and withdrew from everything. I isolated myself and stayed in bed most days. All I wanted to do was sleep because I don't have to think when I sleep. Every minute I was awake was another minute I had the same thoughts just circulating my head. Whenever I looked at my wife and my kids, I felt guilty because I was just getting these unwanted images and thoughts in my mind all day. I couldn't think about anything else or even focus on anything else. It wouldn't just be about them, and I would have thoughts of suicide, imagining myself jumping in front of a wagon, jumping off a bridge, overdosing, hanging myself, cutting my wrists, and slicing my neck. Everything!

But I couldn't stop! I was contemplating all day, every day, I lost my self-identity in all this, I developed depersonalization disorder, I lost hope, motivation, objectives/goals, confidence, self-esteem, and worst of all, I felt nothing! Feelingless! Emptiness, no love, no happiness, or anything! I felt like I was already dead!

After a few days of this, I lost it and took the work van. I drove up a motorway for two hours, ruminating about how I would end my life, and people were ringing me. I was ignoring them all! Forty/Fifty calls were missed. I contemplated driving off the motorway into the bridge or a tree. I was thinking, 'do I pull over and just jump off the bridge? But in the end, I decided to drive to my son's grave and end my life there.

I drove two hours back home and sat outside my son's graveyard in the van. I was thinking of piping from the exhaust into the van or slitting my wrists. I went with the latter, and I decided to do it. My anxiety was through the roof because of what I was about to do, but deep down, I was scared. I didn't want to do this, but I also didn't want to continue living with these thoughts. This was easier even though it was still hard. I sat in the driver's seat with the blades in my hand, ready to cut myself and hope it ended my life, but deep down, I didn't want this. I looked around in the dark, hoping someone might stop me, so it looked like I was going to do it, but someone caught me just in time! I looked in my mirror and saw a white car pull up behind me down the road, and there it was. My friends came! They opened the door and chucked the blade out of my hand, and I just broke down and cried!

The days didn't get any easier. Every day I was dealing with this same s**t. The thoughts about me, the thoughts about other people, they just kept coming and coming and coming. I couldn't stop them. I didn't know how to or if there was a way to. Every day, I tried to get reassurance from people to tell me I was safe, but that didn't last long.

The reassurance you need today isn't the same as tomorrow, and you need more and more... when that ran out, I would try different ways. I web searched everything I felt, everything I saw and tried self-diagnosing. That didn't work either because I always diagnosed myself with numerous different disorders. This didn't help me any further because I would find one article that reassured me and another that would make me question everything repeatedly and spike my anxiety, bouncing in and out of reassurance. I was all over the place with this. I was heavily depressed and severely anxious, seeking to find answers to hopefully relieve this problem because I just wanted it to end. Then to top it all off, two months later, we were hit with COVID19. This added to the stress, the anxiety and the fear of the unknown, which kept circulating and feeding everything else. I was scared that my whole life was about to flip upside down.

Imagine waking up every day feeling sick to the stomach with anxiety overdrive, feeling like you've got another mental battle with your thoughts again, feeling lost, lonely, and numb. It gives you no hope and instantly drives more intrusive thoughts, which you seem to thrive on, fueling the fire that won't die down but only grows. It's exhausting.

Everyday! The thoughts created this anxiety that then would produce physical feelings like urges and twitching in your arms and legs, the racing heartbeat, the racing mind, the mental and physical restlessness, the need to move but didn't want to be anywhere, pacing through the room to room and how do you hide it all? How do you stop someone else from seeing that, so they don't ask you if you're okay? Because if they do, it makes it real! It makes it known that you're not okay and you're still going through the same stuff months later, and you aren't dealing with it!

Certain people did not help when I was going through this, and I don't blame them because how hard must it be trying to help someone without knowing what help they need or fully understanding what it is they're going through, what it is they're feeling? It's difficult; therefore, mental health is so hard to deal with. It's a personal experience that causes isolation. I didn't observe this at the time because I only cared about getting better.

I remember a family member coming to my house once to see us. They first, said to me, "you, okay? Are you still having their voices"? This infuriated me, made me anxious, and repeatedly questioned everything. Everything I had researched or been told in my time trying to deal with this just disappeared, all I thought about was 'voices'. Are they voices? Oh, my god! Voices! 'I'm going crazy! I've got voices! My anxiety, yet again, was out of control, and it triggered everything all over again. I was panicking and trying to show that I was fine and strong. Asserting reinforcement from my side, I just replied, "What do you mean voices?" They're not voices" Then I'd spend the next fifteen minutes explaining and trying to justify to them what it was I was going through so that they didn't think I had 'voices. Which I wasn't sure about. I was mentally fragile, so guess what happened next...

Yes, you guessed it! Back onto the reassurance train, I went. I researched my disorder, all other disorders, and what it was like to hear voices because I needed to reassure myself that it wasn't voices and that I wasn't going crazy! I can't reiterate how scary this was for me, going through this all on my own, knowing that nobody could help me, and that's what I needed... HELP! I was weak, and I was empty, I was scared, I was lonely, I was sticky! My mind would stick to anything that anyone said, and I would question it to then have to seek reassurance.

CHAPTER FOUR: FINDING HELP

After months, with no help from the mental health service and long waiting times, I took it upon myself to find help elsewhere. The company I worked for had an employee assistance program, and I took advantage of this benefit. However, they didn't recognize the help I needed for the problem I was faced with, I attended ten sessions, and all I got was someone to talk to but no direction of when this was going to be dealt with or in my mind when this was going to end. The sessions were great for talking to someone about my issues and thoughts, but when it came to an understanding and what help I needed, there was a lack of support in that area. I then paid for a private therapist, leading to the same conclusions. I was losing hope/faith that I would ever recover from this, and the only endpoint was the one I nearly allowed myself to do just a short while before. My emotions were still in disarray. I was frustrated and angry and began realizing that maybe the only way was for me to get myself out of this, but I didn't know what I was going through or dealing with, so how was I supposed to do that? Again, sparking thoughts of suicide seemed to be the daily thought process.

The next and what felt to be the last option in finding help from someone else was when I spoke to a work colleague about what I was going through, and I talked about it gently as I was cautious about how others would react or perceive what I was saying to them.

A short while into the conversation, I began to unveil that he has and does experience the same things from time to time, but it didn't seem to be from the same level I had. He is also very sensitive, wearing his heart on his sleeve like myself. The conversation led to me finding out that his family member is a mental health therapist, and she works privately, and I began to find out more and later in that month, my company offered to pay the therapist for ten sessions for me to go through.

Whilst waiting for the therapy to start, I researched online some more and found out that I was closer to an answer than I had been waiting what seemed to be forever to get close to one. The symptoms that I was getting close to was OCD, which was orientated around harm, known as 'Harm OCD' the therapy required for this is part of CBT therapy, which stands for Cognitive Behavioral Therapy. Part of that program consists of ERP, Exposure and Response Therapy. It was a massive relief knowing that I was somewhat closer to help and an answer, but such a long way off a cure, well, if a cure existed for what I had developed.

My therapy started a few weeks later, and I could talk about everything and get responses that made me feel like the therapist understood, as this was key. Having no confidence in your therapist is no help when you're struggling with something mentally. This was great, and my mood started lifting through lockdowns. I was reading more books, engaging with people more and trying to enjoy every day. Even when I still had these sorts of thoughts running through my head, it was still horrible but livable. The ten sessions ended, and I felt I had enough knowledge to fight this. I had a lot of information and read many books to understand how the brain works and everything. Well, that was easier said than done.

Over the next few months in lockdown, I tried every day to fight this, using advice from professionals and advice online, but it seemed only to work temporarily. I would start every day with a hard slog of getting myself out of bed and trying to find the motivation to fight this again. It takes a lot of emotional energy to keep your mind levelheaded, but I kept trying and trying. It seemed to be working in lockdown, and I was still employed, so I didn't have a lot of stress to deal with during the COVID period.

I would go maybe one or two days and then fall back down again, and then I would go a week and then fall back down again. I kept questioning my feelings every day, 'why don't I feel anything? I felt helpless but frustrated and angry that I was allowing myself to let this happen as if it were my fault. I thought it was my fault, but the therapists told me it was not. It was very confusing for me, but I was confused anyway, so what did it matter?

The help I got and the research I had done has gotten me this far, but nothing is left out there. This is how I felt!

That is where I believe most mental health disorders lead, as all my mental health experiences have led me to this, to the point of looking down a long tunnel with no light at the end, hoping that a miracle will come along and take all the pain away. But, as you can imagine, and I am sorry to say, this is further than reality because no miracle will come and take it away from you.

You must find the inner strength to pick yourself back up and fight another day. The amount of emotional draining, the tiredness, the weaknesses buried within your mind and physicality, and the doubts is all part of it, but you must sit with it. The quicker you get used to being comfortable being uncomfortable, the better. I also know how suffocating it is when you're going through this. The feeling of feeling alone even when you're in a room full of people, the sense of feeling restless, the heavy gut feeling for hours and days from all the anxiety that is being created within but guess what! It's not forever!

In moments like this, you literally must cherish the good, embrace the negative feelings or, in this case, embrace feeling empty because it is short-lived. The only reason you think empty is the stress and trauma you are in or under. The brain switches certain parts of its functionality down when you have high-stress levels, which it does because it needs to survive! You wouldn't think about what shopping you'd need from a supermarket if faced with a bear standing in front of you! This is the same, and the anxiety comes because you have told your brain that there is danger, whether in a thought, a physical being, or in a situation you fear.

I wrote this chapter for you, the reader. Because I have been through this, I know this, but I am here for you. Feel my words comfort you as you read. I have felt rock bottom, and I am sitting with you now. If you're feeling confused, it's okay! If you are feeling lost, it's okay! If you're feeling alone, it's okay! It is not forever! Believe me! If I can get through this, so can you! Just be brave and get used to feeling uncomfortable for a while!

CHAPTER FIVE: UNDERSTANDING THE OCD DIAGNOSIS

L et's look at specifically was OCD is. It stands for obsessive-compulsive disorder.

Obsessive thoughts can interrupt your daily life, upsetting you and making it hard to do things you want to do. Even if you're aware they aren't real and know you won't act on them, you may still feel distressed and worry you could act on them. As a result, you might try to avoid everything that triggers these thoughts.

Compulsions refer to mental or physical responses or behaviors to obsessions. You may need to repeat these behaviors even though you don't want to be doing them. This can take up hours of your day. Carrying out these compulsions brings about a sense of relief from an obsession, but this feeling is usually short-lived. And disorder just means anything that appears to be out of control. Sometimes compulsions are related and relevant to an obsession. For example, you might check, unlock, and relock your front door seven times before leaving to prevent a break-in.

In general, most people with OCD experience an obsessive thought and then feel compelled to perform an action or compulsion to help relieve the anxiety or stress associated with the obsession. Below are a few different types of OCD.

Contamination is probably the most stereotyped form of OCD. People affected by this fear getting sick or infecting someone they care about after encountering serious bacteria.

Perfectionist is a little different in that it's difficult to identify a specific fear underlying it. Instead, it's usually more like a strong feeling that something isn't right when things aren't done in a certain way.

Relationships leave people completely unable to tolerate the uncertainty of intimate relationships, giving them obsessions about the "rightness" of their relationship and the countless other possibilities that daily life brings.

Harm causes people to be deeply disturbed by the violent or what's known as intrusive thoughts that just about everyone has experienced. While most people can shrug off these thoughts, those with harmful OCD can become completely overwhelmed by them.

Sexual orientation involves obsessions about one's sexuality. It's often called homosexual OCD, but this is misleading. It can happen to people of any sexuality, about any other sexuality.

When I got told what I was suffering from, I didn't understand it, and I always thought OCD was a good thing because people always laughed and joked about having 'cleaning OCD'. I never perceived this to be a bad thing, and it's the only thing I heard anyone relate OCD too. I never heard anyone say, 'I've got harm OCD' and started laughing and joking or 'I've got religious OCD and start laughing and joking or even 'homosexual OCD' and start laughing and joking.

People fail to understand the complexity of OCD and how it makes people feel, like imagine not doing something because you fear the afterwards or imagine doing something you don't want to do because you want to feel reassured or relieved! When I was younger, I used to not step on cracks on the ground or walk under signs or ladders, or I'd have to not leave things on odd numbers because if I did, I was scared something bad would happen! I still do these today; I must check everything repeatedly because I'm scared of what might happen if I don't check it right.

Harm OCD(Pure-O) is often dealing with obsessive thinking and or engaging in compulsive behaviour to reduce the anxiety associated with these thoughts, such as fear of causing harm to yourself or others, Intrusive thoughts of engaging in violence against yourself or others, Self-doubt regarding whether you will act on obsessive thoughts, Avoidance behaviours (compulsions) to prevent violence against self or others.

The different compulsions range depending on what type of OCD you have, and they are all mostly physical in one way or another. Harm OCD is mostly mental but still has physical compulsions, such as researching the web for reassurance.

The thoughts grabbed me; if I washed the pots, I would avoid touching the knives. If my wife was cooking, I would stay away from the knife. I was terrified. I would drive, and I'd get thought of me driving off the road into pedestrians or not braking around a corner and driving straight off the road;

These thoughts seemed to be about everything I didn't want to think about and most of the time, they would be about the people that was closest to me in my life.

OCD isn't just the problem, though. I developed GAD, which stands for General Anxiety Disorder, which is also quite common to have both simultaneously. GAD causes you to feel anxious about a wide range of situations and issues rather than one specific theme or obsession, so the anxiety created can often lead to a misdiagnosis of OCD in people. When you throw anxiety in the mix, it becomes toxic.

In my experience, it becomes a vicious circle between stress, anxiety, and depression and these all feed on each other, so you must break the loop sooner rather than later.

What is hard for people to understand that goes through this is that the brain is doing the reverse of what you think it is doing. Very clever, you may say, or do you say, "why am I letting myself go through this" just like I did for years? It's very hard to understand what is happening to you when you are going through it, but when you start learning and understanding what is happening, you can start to make some sort of sense.

Let me run you through a quick situation to explain what I mean. Imagine you had a thought pop in your head like I did, just like everyone has, which is around 50,000 per day, so a few stats have said in the past. Let's say that out of the 50,000, you had a few weird ones that popped up like, I don't know, maybe you were talking to someone at work, and you thought, 'I hope they don't spit on me whilst they are talking, or a quite common one would be sitting at a train platform and having the thought of 'pushing someone onto the track', or you're on a balcony with someone, and you get a thought that looks something like 'imagine if they fell off or 'you throwing them off. These are all intrusive thoughts because intrusive thought is any unwanted thoughts that can pop into our heads without warning at any time. Now you see what I mean. Anybody and everybody get them, it's what's perceived as 'normal' some may not recognize them, and some may do. Still, the biggest difference is that anyone with OCD will question their thoughts and latch onto them because they fear them. Just like I did, and that wears the disorder starts in chapter three.

Many people say the brain is clever and it's the most fascinating and powerful thing in life. I don't disagree in many ways; I believe when it is used for the right things, it can do a lot for you. We've gone through generations forever changing and advancing in ways nobody would have ever believed, so yes, it is clever! But, in this instance, you question why something so clever can create something like this.

What happens with OCD is that you develop it in many ways. I believe it is still unknown what the true cause of OCD is, but many articles say that it is developed in various ways. Genetics, brain abnormalities, and the environment, such as stress, play a role. It often starts in teens or early adulthood. Some people with OCD have areas of unusually high activity in their brain or low levels of a chemical called serotonin.

So, once you develop OCD, the disorder starts feeding on certain themes such as sexual, harm etc. The thoughts come in, you see the thought, it has some sort of fear, and you tell your brain the thought is dangerous. It stores this, where you get something called thought-action fusion, where it fuses the thought and feeling together. Therefore, when you get the same thought or another one of similar themes, you get an automatic response, the conscious mind doesn't see the thought until it has come to the forefront. Still, the subconscious mind has already recognized it.

The more anxious you get, the more difficult it is to deal with this thought and any others it produces. The brain has started shutting certain parts down because of the stress. It thinks you are in danger. It's waiting for a response from you, and if you don't react with a certain thought that scared you, it sends another one that's either the same or within the same theme, although sometimes it can switch themes to trigger a response from you. I have also had it where it will throw into my dreams, but it is quite uncommon.

CHAPTER SIX: STEPS TO RECOVERY POST JOURNEY

You may be wondering why I call this disorder a mental health "journey" I call it a journey because, in my opinion, it is ongoing with different stages. It's how we evaluate the different effects that help us manage them better to give every chance of recovery.

Once I understood what I was dealing with, it wasn't any easier because I knew that there was only me that is going to get myself out of this situation, and that's why I still have the odd setback now and again, because I am still dealing with it, and I am human. You must understand that trying to retrain the brain to do something different when you've done the same for years isn't going to be easy, and that's why it isn't a short process.

As I mentioned, you get a thought with these specific thoughts, tell your brain it is dangerous, and then put yourself into an anxious state. Depending how you react depends on how far you go. As I did with a lack of knowledge and the level of questioning and rumination, I went all the way. It didn't stop for a long time; throughout the process, it stripped everything from me, especially my confidence, self-esteem, self-worth and self-identity. Going from telling your brain that thought is dangerous, or it means something, to telling it the same thought isn't dangerous and means nothing is very confusing. You must maintain consistency through the recovery process.

Disregarding thoughts is the best way to recover from OCD. By disregarding, I mean you must acknowledge them but don't ruminate. Don't find a meaning for them, and they're intrusive thoughts. They mean nothing to you.

Thinking about something doesn't make it more likely that it will happen, nor does it make you a bad person for a thought you are not in control of! People asked me if I was putting my name in this book, and I questioned it. Did I question why? This is my story: I didn't choose to have OCD, I didn't choose to have those thoughts, I didn't choose to hit rock bottom. I chose how to react because that is the only thing I am in control of!!

You need to track your ruminations. If you're struggling to get out of bed because you're contemplating, guess what! Get up and get on with your day, rumination will bury you, and you will not find any answers! Accept it and move on. Accept the thought and choose to disregard it. You're in control. You choose what you want to spend time thinking about. If you struggle, allocate time, like saying, "I'll spend 30 minutes later thinking about that", but you must be disciplined. If you let it take hold, then you will slow recovery.

Nobody is perfect. You will have setbacks when it gets hard. If something in your life causes more stress, then you're going to be more vulnerable and fragile, you may not have the strength to deal with the OCD that day, but that's fine! Do it the next day, and there is no pressure. Recovery takes as long as it takes. I believe you can do it! Just keep pushing forward!

I am not ashamed, and I am not guilty. I am not empty, I am Sean Bell, and I have good and bad experiences with mental health. I am aware of mental health disorders; I have chosen to become educated on how mental health can affect lives, and I CHOSE to share it with you! I chose to share it with you because I care more about trying to help anyone else that may not know what they're going through and how it might affect them than how I may look in someone else eyes or someone else's opinion that quite frankly doesn't matter! It doesn't matter because they don't know what it's like! And if they did, they wouldn't be judgmental!

EPILOGUE/CONCLUSION

I hope my story in this book has helped you because that's why I wrote it. I struggled and still struggle with my mental health some days. I have accepted that it's okay not to be okay, but at the same time, you must control it. You are your person, you have your own life, and you will find your way to manage whatever you have to deal with in life but know this! There is always someone out there that will look out for you, and there is always someone out there that has been through whatever it is you are going through. You need to reach out, and you are not alone! I want this book to represent how you can get out of what seems to be a very dark place, and you can't get any lonelier than in your world! If you need to talk, please get in touch with someone like I did. I didn't stop until I found answers. Speak to friends/family, your local healthcare service, and GP. Mental health awareness is becoming more known with more research and techniques to deal with different disorders.